Qigong:

Foundation Practices

Twelve Health Exercises from the
Wah Family System

By John Munro

ii

Note

No part of this book is intended as medical advice, or to be used as a substitute for appropriate medical care.

Neither this nor any other exercise program should be followed without first consulting a health care professional. If you have any special conditions requiring attention, you should consult with your health care professional regarding the suitability of the exercises and practices contained in this book and possible modifications.

The author and publisher are not liable for any damage, injury or other adverse outcome resulting from the application of information contained in this book.

ISBN 978-0-473-14339-8

Published by Infosource Ltd
Auckland
New Zealand

Cover design by John Munro
Cover design © 2008 John Munro

To my mother,
for her patience and encouragement.

·d

The book you are about to read is authored by one of my best students, with the best intentions in mind. This book is only an introduction to the extent of the practices involved in Chi Kung (Qigong), and by no means claims to be the best or most original. It is however my sincere wish that it will be of assistance to enthusiasts of exercise, be they martial artists or non martial artists. This book should be looked on and used as a reference and combined with competent tuition from a suitably qualified instructor.

The exercises you see in this book are derived from movements used in the Wah gar system. Movements of this type have been used for thousands of years and are not the sole domain of the Wah gar system. These exercises, and variations of them, are common to many other family styles of Kung Fu and Chi Kung, which also use them for building up energy and vitality.

If after reading this fine book you decide to take up Chi Kung practice, then the book and the author have done their job.

There is no exercise system on the planet that could benefit you more than Chi Kung, filling you with vitality and energy and at the same time improving your health and chances of living a long and productive life. This book is the first step for you in understanding the simplicity and availability of the system.

There is no reason why everyone shouldn't take up this sort of exercise, young and old. If you take up the practice of Chi Kung then your life will change for the good and forever. I am not all that far from 80 years of age now and I still practice as often as I can - and I still work seven days a week, up to twelve hours a day. Chi Kung has supported me mentally and physically throughout my adult life, I simply cannot recommend the exercise enough to you.

The principles of practice and philosophy of Chi Kung have marched proudly down through ages, right to the present day. Join in the march and change your life. Be fit and active and enjoy good mental and physical health all your life.

I know that you, the person reading this book, will enjoy many of the exercises offered. As you work your way through it, you, or people you know, will benefit greatly from what is presented. You are now challenged to start today to put into action the practices of Chi Kung.

The bell has rung; get into the ring and fight to change your life.

DR ALASTAIR LAUBACH-BOURNE.

Note on spelling and pronunciation:

Over the years there have been a number of systems for translating Chinese words into the English alphabet. For this reason you will see many different spellings of the same terms. Qigong can variously be spelt: Qigong, Chi Kung, Chi Gung, Chi Gong and so on. Rest assured, even though the spellings look quite different, they are actually all talking about the same thing. The first word or part of the word, 'Qi' or 'Chi' means energy or breath. The second word or part of the word, 'Gong', 'Kung' or 'Gung' means work or skill.

In more recent years the Pinyin system of spelling has been developed and is now the official method of the People's Republic of China. The spelling 'Qigong' comes from this system. It is this spelling that will be used throughout the book.

The word 'Qi' is pronounced "chee" as in cheese.
The word 'Gong' is pronounced "gong" as in a hanging metal disk, which you hit to make a noise.

Table of Contents

xiv

Introduction

For thousands of years the Chinese have had a secret. A secret that has allowed them to treat illness in its earliest stages, a secret that allows athletes to perform amazing seemingly superhuman feats of strength and agility, a secret that promises a long and healthy life to those who understand and apply it. The secret is that rather than focusing purely on the physical elements of the body, the muscles, bones, blood and so on, they focus on the subtle energy running through the body. This is the energy that quickens the muscles, directs the formation of the bones and causes the blood to perform its proper function. It is responsible for all the physical functions and structures of the body. By paying attention to the state of this energy and making sure that there is an adequate supply circulating freely through the body, physical problems are avoided virtually before they start.

This energy, called qi, is the basis for Chinese medicine and the key to the power of Chinese martial arts. Qigong is the method of strengthening this energy and directing it through the body. Medically qigong has been shown to help with conditions including asthma, back pain, cancer, drug addiction, hypertension, low immune system, low bone density, poor balance, senility, poor sexual function, stress, stroke and many other conditions. The studies are numerous and the evidence is sound. To go into all the conditions that qigong is helpful for would require a book in itself. If you are interested in specific details of the benefits of qigong for a particular condition, there are many excellent resources on the internet which can help you. You can rest assured though, that whatever the condition - qigong is likely to be of assistance, because good qigong practice is not only about improving specific conditions, but building up energy and vitality in the whole body which will then allow natural healing to take place. Just a few minutes a day can help not only to recover from such conditions, but to prevent them from occurring in the first place.

The secret of qigong is a secret no longer. Qigong is beginning to be taught throughout the western world. You will have seen people practicing in parks early in the morning. You may have seen shows on TV exploring the amazing feats accomplished by its practitioners; you may have even noticed it popping up on the group fitness schedule at your local gym. Qigong is suitable for all ages and stages of life. In my classes I find older people coming to preserve and improve their health, the middle aged coming to de-stress, and the young coming to develop athletic prowess. As an exercise system it develops strength, flexibility and cardiovascular fitness all at the same time, while also providing mental refreshment as you take time out from the hustle, bustle and stresses of modern living.

It is my belief that qigong offers benefits like no other system of exercise. This book is part of my contribution to sharing these wonderful benefits with the world.

Those of you that have practiced other qigong forms will notice that some of the exercises in this book are familiar, some not so. Qigong exercises have been practiced for thousands of years and different styles choose different sets as their foundation for health and wellbeing.

There is no great mystery to qigong exercises, different movements twist, stretch, bend and stimulate different areas of the body. This combined with mental focus affects the flow of energy in the body. The exercises in this book have been organized into a set on the basis of their action on the internal organs and major meridians of Chinese medicine. Each exercise provides specific benefit to one of the twelve organ/meridian systems of Chinese medicine, and when practiced as a set they provide benefit to the whole body in a safe, gentle and balanced way.

This book is by no means an exhaustive analysis of the theory and application of qigong. It is intended primarily as a How-To for this basic set of qigong exercises. These exercises will provide you with a firm foundation for your health and for further qigong study if you wish to pursue this ancient secret in greater depth.

Chapter One: History of Qigong

Various inscriptions and ancient writings dating back thousands of years have been found which refer to qigong, giving evidence of its ancient origins. To some extent however qigong's origins have been lost in the mists of time. While the ancient writings refer to qigong, they generally do not give a very complete description of the practices. This is due to the secrecy that often surrounded qigong. Qigong practices were found to have so great benefit, that those who knew them would keep them to themselves to give them the advantage over others.

Historically qigong was associated closely with Chinese medicine, the martial arts and even religion. The details of practices were closely guarded secrets that were passed on in person to only a few trusted students. The Chinese doctor who developed a reputation for his healing skill did not want his competitors to learn his methods or they might take away his customers. The martial artist wanted to preserve every advantage over his opponent, as it might mean the difference between life and death. The monk would only pass on the deep knowledge of how to further develop the mind and body to a few who had proven themselves worthy. Often the secrets to a qigong system were passed on only to immediate family members.

The practices that various systems used were diverse, ranging from still meditations, to making various special sounds with the voice, bells and other objects, to vigorous dances and so on. Anything that increases and strengthens the energy or develops skill with using energy can properly be considered a form of qigong. The most common type of qigong practiced was slow graceful moving exercises often based on the movements of wild animals, or simple activities that people would perform day to day. Peasants found that if they performed these movements they became sick less often, and if they were already sick they recovered faster. Martial artists found that by modifying the exercises somewhat they developed great strength and resilience, and with enough dedicated practice they were able to develop unusual abilities. Medical doctors found that they could give certain exercises to their patients for specific conditions to speed up the healing process. They also found that by regular practice themselves; they could improve their healing abilities. Monks, whose lifestyles were based on prolonged periods of sitting meditation, found that they would become weak and less alert over a period of time. Performing these exercises maintained the health of their bodies and minds.

Various sets of these exercises were developed over thousands of years. A master would practice the exercises and pass them on to his students. Sometimes the students would not remember them properly and start doing them differently, or the student would find that by making small changes they got better results. Other times masters having developed sufficient understanding would create whole new sets of exercises to better suit their purposes and help to develop abilities they thought were valuable for them and their students, whether they be martial, medical or religious.

So in our present day you will often see sets of exercises taught claiming to be from some very ancient origin. You will then see someone else teaching another very different set of exercises claiming to come from the same ancient origin. Is one of them right and one of them wrong? Is one lying and the other telling the truth? Probably not. They may both be right and truthful. The exercises have just evolved and developed as they were passed down through various teachers and students. As such it is best not to worry too much about the exact ancient origin of each exercise, but to strive to understand the principles and gain the benefits contained in the particular version of the exercise you are learning.

My primary qigong training was in the Wah family style. This family's style of kung fu is very hard and aggressive, requiring many years of tough physical training and discipline. The tough physical nature of the style meant that an effective means of relaxing and healing the body was required to overcome injury and ensure a long, healthy, and productive life. This led to a great emphasis on the importance of qigong within the style and the development of a particularly effective system for cultivating and using the body's qi.

As with so many traditional styles, the Wah family style was kept strictly within the family - a very closely kept secret. So how did a westerner like me come to learn it?

Sadly during the Second World War the entire village the family lived in was wiped out by Japanese troops. Fortunately at the time the head of the family, Wah Li Yeung, was involved with training British troops in Burma and survived. Later, having moved to England after the war, Wah Li Yeung found himself an old man with no family members to carry on the thousands of years of accumulated knowledge the style represents. Through a chance meeting on a city street, Wah Li Yeung became impressed with the character of two young

British men. He took them on as his students, training them full time, eight hours a day, for several years so that the style could be carried on after his passing. One of these young British men was Alastair Laubach-Bourne - the current head of the style, the other has since passed away.

For many years Alastair Bourne kept with family tradition and did not teach anyone the style. Then in the seventies he noticed that other Chinese were beginning to openly teach their styles to westerners and Alastair decided to begin teaching as well. I am one of his students.

We are fortunate to live now in a time of new openness about sharing the health and vitality giving secrets qigong has to offer, and to still have living receptacles of this knowledge such as Alastair-Bourne with us to aid our learning. We are on the brink of a renaissance in understanding of qigong. This new openness has cleared the way for millions to practice this ancient art, it has allowed practitioners of different styles to openly learn from and compare with one another, enabling the principles that yield such amazing results to be better understood. The door has also opened for scientific investigation into the mechanisms by which qigong works and exciting progress is being made in this area.

By practicing qigong you are participating in both the preservation of an ancient tradition and also contributing to the evolution of these practices to suit modern day living.

Chapter Two: Principles of Practice

As has been mentioned qigong exercise involves not just the body but the mind as well. It is not interested only in gross physical movements, but in the subtle functioning of the body's systems. For the purposes of these exercises there are four principles that will help in influencing these subtle functions.

These are:

1. Quieting the mind and directing the intention.
2. Correct posture to allow free movement of energy.
3. Regulating the breath to stimulate the energy and influence the body.
4. Awareness of energy

Each of these principles will be the subject of subsequent chapters. You will notice as you read through these chapters that each of these principles influence the others significantly.

Qigong is very efficient in that it gives you the benefit of all these principles at the same time. Instead of having to do a meditation session, a breath work session, a postural correction session, and an energy awareness session, your qigong practice can help you to incorporate and benefit from all of these principles at once.

This can seem difficult at first, as you are changing many habits which you have accumulated over a long time. Reading through these chapters and practicing the exercises in each of them one by one will help you to become skilled in each of these areas before combining them together into your qigong practice.

The final section of this book covers twelve qigong health exercises which together stimulate and strengthen the energy through all the organ systems of your body. There is a brief section on the rationale behind these exercises, followed by in depth instructions on how to perform them.

These exercises work on a number of levels. If you simply perform the movements, they will give you a nice gentle physical workout, loosening your joints and developing your balance and flexibility. As you integrate your breathe and sensory awareness into the movements your posture will begin to improve and you will begin to build up energy in your body. Finally once you have a good sense of the energy flowing in your body you will be able to direct that energy to specific parts of your body and strengthen the various internal organs as you exercise.

It is recommended that you learn two or three of the exercises at a time. Practice them regularly until you are comfortable with them and can remember them easily, and then move on and learn another two or three exercises. In this way you will quickly learn and be able to remember all 12 exercises without having to constantly refer to the book. Once you have learned the movements you can begin to focus more on your breathing and awareness throughout the exercises, greatly increasing the efficiency and efficacy of the exercises.

Finally it is worth noting the importance of regular practice. You will gain some benefit from practicing your qigong even just once a week. Certainly you will learn the physical movements, and over time your awareness of your energy will grow little by little. However, the development of your awareness and energy will be slow. For maximum benefit it is best to practice your qigong every day, or at least four or five times a week if every day is not possible.

In our modern lives filled with stressful situations, bad habits, and unnatural environmental influences, many of us can compare our bodies to a piece of land which is experiencing a drought, a drought of qi or vital energy! We are designed to have a constant flow of qi running like rivers through our bodies. When the rivers are full all the surrounding tissues have a constant supply of life giving, health sustaining qi. When more qi comes in, the tissues are able to use it well, and any excess gently seeps into the rivers to circulate to other areas or to be stored for future use in the lakes and seas. However when the rivers have dried up or are blocked through stress, exposure to pollution, lack of exercise etc, and there is a sudden deluge, the tissues are not able to cope with it all at once and the excess runs off quickly causing the rivers to flood. The body is not able to handle all this qi all at once so it will quickly dissipate, very little will be kept in the cells of the body. It may even make you feel quite unwell.

Far better to do little and often, gradually building up the level of qi in the tissues of your body, over time replenishing the rivers and their normal flow and eventually building up the reservoirs of qi in your body. Your progress will be steady and sure.

It is much better to do ten minutes every day than one hour once a week. Over time you will be able to, and want to, do more. Do so if you wish.

Chapter Three: Quieting the Mind

When we think of a particular object or experience, our bodies will respond in tangible ways, even though we have only thought about it. For example, when we think about our favorite food, (you can try this now if you want, picture your favorite food, it might be a spicy ethnic dish, it might be a certain tangy fruit, it might be chocolate—whatever you really like. Remember the smell, the taste, the texture in your mouth), for many of us our mouths will start to water as our bodies produce saliva ready to start the process of digesting the food, even though we have only thought about it, there is no actual food in front of us. You may even start to have a warm feeling in your tummy as your body directs energy there.

Just as our body responds physically to the thought of food, it will respond to other thoughts that cross our minds. For example if we are thinking about the argument we had with our boss yesterday and how we have to face him again today, our shoulders might tense up, our jaw might clench, our breathing might get more shallow—we might even end up with a headache. All this from just thinking about the situation.

The functions of our bodies are largely directed by our minds, both conscious and unconscious. This goes both for the more obvious functions such as the tension in our muscles, right down to the less discernible ones such as release of hormones, electrical activity and the flow of our qi.

In our busy modern world we have lots of things to think

about. Work, family, interest rates, the price of petrol at the pump. In addition to this we have the media constantly feeding us news about things going on around the world, both good and bad. There is a constant stream of information directed at us which requires our attention; television, the internet, even the music on the radio keeps our minds occupied 24/7. This directs the resources of our bodies in many ways which we are not conscious of, many of which are undesirable.

It is very helpful in our daily lives to take time out from the clutter of all the different thoughts in our minds. This allows the tensions and other patterns we have formed in our body to be released, even if only for a short time. As we get into the habit over time we will release more and more, holding on to less and less unnecessary tension in our bodies during our regular daily activities. This also gives our mind a rest, making it easier to cope with stress and the challenges of our lives.

When our mind is calm, we are able to direct all our body's resources on the task at hand, allowing us to perform tasks more efficiently and with more ease. This will also allow you to become more aware of the subtle functions of your body and begin to become aware of your qi and direct its action.

There are a number of things that will help you to develop this habit of having a quiet mind throughout your qigong practice.

You can begin by practicing some simple meditation techniques alone. This will give you practice working with quieting your mind before you then move on to doing this in conjunction with the moving qigong exercises.

For all of these meditations it is best if you find somewhere quiet where you will not be distracted. If you are at home or work, make sure the phone is turned off so you will not be disturbed. Wear loose comfortable clothing. This may be as simple as taking your belt off and loosening your tie if you wear one, there is no need for special clothing, just make sure you are comfortable with no restrictive pressures on your body. Make sure you are warm enough and that there are no drafts.

You can perform these simple meditations while sitting in a chair, sitting or kneeling on the floor, or even lying down on the floor or a bed. Whatever your position, just make sure you will be comfortable in that position for five, ten or twenty minutes, however long you plan to meditate for.

Meditation One: Breath Awareness

The most basic type of meditation you can do is simple breath awareness. Breathing is something we all do, all the time. It is a simple function we are consciously aware of and can easily put our attention on. By putting our attention on this simple function, and keeping it there for a period of time, we can allow our mind to release the other things it is thinking about and just follow the movement of our breath in and out. This is very calming to our mind, as it is not demanding, and gradually our breath will begin to deepen and relax as our body's resources become focused on it. The rest of our body will also begin to relax as we release the tensions caused by the other things we have been thinking about both consciously and unconsciously.

To do this meditation, simply become aware of the air coming in through your nose. Follow it as it goes down your throat and into your lungs. It will help if you close your eyes so that you can focus fully on your breath. Notice the warmth or coolness of the air. Notice what parts of your body expand and contract through the different phases of your breath. Simply follow your breath, being aware of it for several minutes, noticing your natural pattern of breathing and how it begins to shift, relax and deepen simply by you being aware of it.

After several minutes you can begin to influence the pattern of your breathing consciously to make it even deeper and fuller (Chapter Four: Regulating the Breath will give you more instructions on how you can do this).

You can then begin to work with the rhythm of the breath, counting the length of the inhalation and exhalation and the pauses in between. A rhythm of 8:4:8:4 is an excellent one to aim for. This is the rhythm of the universe. Inhale for eight, pause for four, exhale for eight, pause for four. Ideally the counts are heartbeats. If you are not yet aware enough of your heartbeat to do this, the count can simply be seconds. If this rhythm is too difficult for you, you can try 4:2:4:2 or 6:3:6:3.

You can do this simple meditation as often as you like, it will help to calm your mind and relax your body. It will also help to develop more beneficial breathing habits.

Meditation Two: Sensory Awareness

In this meditation we move from holding our awareness purely on one simple function of our bodies to becoming aware of more of our senses and what is going on around us.

Again we begin by getting comfortable and closing our eyes. In our modern world we have an imbalanced reliance on our sense of sight. It is natural for us to gain a lot of information visually, but then when we begin reading, using the internet, watching television, sitting in classrooms where our primary means of learning is looking at visual presentations, this gets out of balance.

Closing our eyes takes the emphasis off our visual sense, allowing this part of our mind to relax. It can then enhance our other senses, allowing us to use a different set of neural connections. It helps us to literally 'reconnect' with our bodies.

Begin again by becoming aware of your breath. Become aware of the air as it enters through your nostrils and moves down into your lungs. Notice your breath start to deepen and relax.

Now become aware of where your body is supported, on the floor, the chair, the bed or wherever you are. Feel each point of contact. Are the soles of your feet on the floor? Do they feel heavy or light? Is there the same amount of weight resting through your left foot as your right? Are you legs supported, how heavy is the pressure? Your buttocks, your back, your shoulders, your arms and hands, your head, become aware of each point where the weight of your body rests. How comfortable are you? Can you adjust your position so you are more comfortable? How does the weight of you body feel now? Can you feel the clothing on your body? Is it rough? smooth? prickly? soft? Can you feel the movement of the air on your skin? Even in a still room your breath will create currents. Can you feel your heart beating? Can you hear it?

Now start to move your awareness outwards. What can you smell? What can you hear immediately around you? What can you hear a little further away? Things will occur around you as you are meditating, you may hear someone walk past outside, you might hear a lawnmower starting, you may feel a breeze spring up. Just be aware of these things. Notice them, see what else you can feel, hear and smell. Relax in comfort and safety, aware of all you can sense around you.

When it is time for you to finish your meditation bring your awareness right back into your body. Feel the weight of your body supported wherever you are. Feel your toes, maybe wiggle them a little. Feel your legs, give them a little rock side to side, feel your torso and arms and head. Gently start to move your body a little. It may feel a bit like waking up from a deep sleep. When you are ready open your eyes. Take your time and get up when you are ready and go on with your daily activities.

Meditation Three: Directing the Intention

Now you have experience with using your senses in meditation, you can begin to consciously direct your body's resources, your qi, in your meditation.

Begin again by becoming aware of your breath. Be aware of the air as it comes in through your nose and down into your lungs. If you have spent some time doing the breathing exercises in chapter four, you will now be familiar with the inward and outward movement of your lower abdomen during your breathing. Feel the energy from your breath descending down into your lower abdomen. With each breath more energy accumulates there. Continue with this awareness until you have a warm ball of

14

energy in your lower abdomen.

Now move this ball with your mind down your right leg to your right foot. Start at the toes. As you continue to breathe in and out, feel more energy going down to the ball of energy in the toes of your right foot. Feel the toes relax. Move the ball of energy up the foot toward the ankle, pausing at the ankle and feeling it relax. Continue moving the ball of energy up the leg towards the knee, and then the hip, pausing as you go whenever you feel an area is a little tight or uncomfortable. Now move the ball of energy down to the toes of your left foot and up your left leg.

With the ball of energy now at the top of your left leg, move the ball of energy through the area of your groin, then your buttocks, continue up through your lower abdomen, your back, and chest, feeling each area glowing with health as the ball of energy moves through it.

Now move the ball of energy down your left arm, pausing and relaxing the shoulder, then the elbow, the wrist, the hand and fingers. Move the ball of energy back up the left arm and down the right, pausing again and loosening each area as you go.

Bring the ball of energy back to your neck, move it slowly up to your head, move it through over your scalp, and over each part of your face, pausing as you go. Now move the ball of energy into your brain and down the centre of your body to your lower abdomen. Let the ball of energy rest there for awhile before you end your meditation.

This is a simple meditation for directing your energy into areas of your body. If you have particular parts of your body that are sore, or you have some sort of problem with, you can focus particularly on these areas. If you have knowledge of anatomy you can also direct the energy quite specifically to organs and even specific glands in your body that you know need attention.

These three simple meditations will give you good practice at quieting your mind, becoming aware of your senses and directing your intention.

When it comes to your qigong practice there are several other things you can do that will help.

Location

It is nice if you can do your qigong outside in a beautiful natural environment, perhaps by a mountain, lake or sea, or even just in a local park. The natural surroundings can help to get our minds out of our day to day activities and on to the natural functioning of our bodies. If this is not possible, your living room, bedroom, office or some other indoor location will be fine. Try to find somewhere clear of clutter where you are unlikely to be distracted. Wherever you go, it is important that you are warm enough and out of direct hot sunlight. Later as you become more accustomed to quieting your mind the conditions around you will not be so important, as you will be less easily distracted.

Time

It is helpful to develop a routine. Find a time that you can practice every day and keep to it as much as possible. Also allow enough time for your practice. DO NOT RUSH. It took me a long time to learn this lesson. Even as I was performing the movements slowly, internally I would be rushing wanting to get through a certain amount, or to move on to other things. It is better to relax and enjoy your practice, just doing as much as you have time for. It is better to relax and really focus and enjoy five minutes of practice of a few exercises than to rush through a whole lot in twenty minutes.

Acceptance

Accept wherever you are at with your qigong practice. Never force anything. Don't breathe or perform the movements more slowly than you are comfortable with, this will only cause more tension in your body and mind. If you have tensions in your body, acknowledge them and work towards making your posture more comfortable. Do not persist if it becomes too uncomfortable, you will make better progress by just going to your own level of comfort and then going a little further next time. When you are doing the energy awareness exercises in Chapter Six, do not try to convince yourself you are feeling more than you are. Just be aware of what you do (or don't) feel and accept it. With time and practice your awareness will grow.

Preparation

If you are able to, it is great if you can do a meditation session before you begin your qigong practice. If not, it is helpful to at least pause for a few moments and become aware of your breath before you begin your practice. This will let your mind clear of the activities of the day and the demands on your attention. It is best not to try to force your mind to be calm and peaceful – it will resist! Just allow the thoughts to surface, but do not follow them. Have you ever noticed when presenting to a group, at the beginning often everyone will be talking to each other and there may be quite a bit of noise, but if you just stand quietly at the front ready to begin, gradually the noise will die off until there is complete silence. This is a good approach to take for calming your own mind. If your mind refuses to be calm, perhaps there is something else you need to attend to? Put your Qigong aside and come back to it another time.

Chapter Four: Regulating The Breath

The Chinese character for qi tells us a lot about the process of developing our energy and increasing our skill with it. The character looks like this:

The character is composed of two parts. The symbol for breath:

Which sits above the symbol for rice or grain:

A simple interpretation of this character is 'steam rising from a cooking pot of rice' - or energy. This fits well with our scientific understanding of how we generate energy in our bodies. We take in food, and in most parts of the world a major part of that food intake will be grain of some sort. That food is digested and the resulting compounds are mixed with oxygen from the air we breathe to release energy wherever we need it in our bodies. So it is not surprising that exercising our abdominal organs and breathing effectively are central to qigong practice.

There are many different types of breathing used in different types of qigong. Each one has different benefits and is useful in its place. Here we will cover some of the simplest ones which will help you with these exercises. The first one we will look at is Buddhist or abdominal breathing.

When this type of breathing is referred to as 'Buddhist breathing' it has nothing to do with the Buddhist religion. It is simply that the Buddhist related traditions tend to use this type of breathing more than others. This is the type of breathing most commonly used by some martial arts, particularly those with a Buddhist connection, and it is also the type of breathing most commonly used in yoga. It is referred to as abdominal breathing because the emphasis is very much on the movement of the lower abdomen.

This type of breathing relies almost entirely on the movement of the diaphragm muscle. The diaphragm muscle forms a dome shape up under our rib cage. When it contracts, it pulls downwards, creating a vacuum which draws air into the lungs, particularly the lower lungs. This downward motion also puts pressure on the digestive organs in the lower abdomen and causes the belly to expand outwards. When the diaphragm muscle relaxes, it pulls back upwards causing air to be expelled from the lungs and the belly to draw back inwards.

This type of breathing is excellent to learn as it emphasizes the use of our diaphragm muscle which is our primary breathing muscle. Many of us have got into habits of breathing mainly into our upper chests and do not regularly use our diaphragm muscle effectively. This breathing also massages the digestive organs in the lower abdomen with the inward and outward movement of the belly.

Breathing Exercise One: Buddhist or Abdominal Breathing

To perform Buddhist breathing, assume a comfortable position, whether this is seated, kneeling, standing or lying on your back. It helps to put one hand on your belly and one on your chest so you can more easily feel what is going on. As you breathe in through your nose, gently allow your belly to extend out. As you breathe out through your nose, gently draw it back in. You should feel with your hands that it is mainly only your belly which is moving in and out, there should be very little movement of your chest.

Repeat for several inhalations and exhalations to get the feel of this type of breathing.

The next type of breathing we will look at is called Daoist or Reverse breathing.

Again the reference to Daoism in the name of this breathing has nothing to do with religion, other than that the Daoists used this type of breathing more than others. It is referred to as reverse breathing because the movement of the abdomen is the opposite of the Buddhist breathing we have just looked at, and the opposite we would expect given the function of the diaphragm muscle. This is the type of breathing most commonly used in some of the Daoist influenced martial arts, and also the type of breathing most commonly used in Pilates.

This type of breathing emphasizes the secondary breathing muscles far more, particularly the intercostal muscles between the ribs. As we breathe in the belly is drawn in, meaning the intercostals muscles have to contract to expand the ribcage and draw it upwards, increasing the space within the ribcage, creating a vacuum and causing air to be drawn into the lungs. As we breath out the belly is extended causing the intercostals to have to lengthen to let the ribcage sink in and downwards expelling the air from the lungs.

This type of breathing is excellent in that it helps us to develop skill with our secondary breathing muscles and develop great strength in them. It is an excellent type of breathing for strenuous physical exertion as the deep core muscles of the lower abdomen work in conjunction with the muscles of the upper torso around the ribcage to provide a strong stable base for the limbs to work from.

Breathing Exercise Two: Daoist Breathing

Again assume a comfortable position whether sitting, kneeling, standing or lying down. Place one hand on your belly, the other on your chest so that you can more easily feel the expansion and contraction of the different parts of your body.

As you inhale through your nose, draw your belly in and feel your chest rise. As you exhale through your mouth expand your belly out and feel your chest fall.

Repeat for several inhalations and exhalations to get the feel of this type of breathing.

The next type of breathing we will look at is Accentuated Natural Breathing.

When we breathe fully and naturally, we use all of the breathing muscles so that we can perform this function most efficiently. Many of us have got into habits whereby we use only a portion of our breathing muscles through only a portion of their range of movement. This greatly reduces the efficiency of our breathing and reduces our overall breathing capacity. We want our breathing to be as efficient as possible, and to have access to our full breathing capacity so that we can go about our activities in life with the greatest ease and grace.

Each of the preceding two exercises has emphasized a portion of the breathing muscles, and they are a great place to start out. The next type of breathing will use ALL the breathing muscles and breath capacity to their fullest extent. Once you have mastered this type of breathing, when you go back to the other types of breathing it will feel like you are only taking half a breath. But first we will need to develop even more skill with our diaphragm and secondary breathing muscles by doing the following exercise.

Breathing Exercise Three: Developing Skill with the Breathing Muscles

For this exercise, again assume a comfortable position whether sitting, kneeling, standing or lying down. Place one hand on your belly, the other on your chest so that you can more easily feel the expansion and contraction of the different parts of your body. Take a full breath in through the nose, pulling the belly in as for Daoist breathing. Now hold the breath and move the belly in and out, in and out. Do this quite rapidly. As the belly moves out the chest will fall, as the belly moves back in the chest will rise. It should feel like there is a bubble moving up and down for your chest to your belly. Move the bubble up and down as many times as you are comfortable, then pull the belly back in and breathe out through the mouth.

Take a few normal relaxed breaths and then repeat the process again several times.

This exercise helps us to gain more conscious control of our diaphragm and secondary breathing muscles. For some of you this may be quite uncomfortable to begin with, but it will become easier with practice. You are also helping to stretch the breathing muscles so you will be able to use a greater portion of their range of motion in your breathing.

I do not recommend you do this type of exercise more than once a day. Over time it will become unnecessary for you to continue to do this exercise as you will begin to fully use your breathing muscles automatically in your daily activities. When we breathe naturally to our full capacity, the movement will begin with the diaphragm pulling down and pushing the belly out. This fills the lower portion of our lungs. Once these are full the middle and upper portions of the ribcage needs to expand to allow the upper portions of the lungs to fill fully. This requires the secondary breathing muscles to contract, expanding the rib cage and lifting it upwards. As this happens the belly will naturally pull back in.

Then as we breathe out the chest will fall and the ribcage relaxes, the belly will extend back out. As we continue to exhale, the diaphragm will relax back upwards expelling the air from the lower portion of the lungs and pulling the belly back in.

This is a natural pattern of breathing. If you stay relaxed when you are exerting yourself very hard, you may notice yourself naturally going into this pattern of breathing, as your body needs to use as much of your breath capacity as possible. Unfortunately for most of us the bad, partial, breathing habits we have developed have become so deeply ingrained that it takes some training for us to regain this natural pattern. In our day to day activities we generally do not need to regularly use our full breath capacity, but learning to use it will give us skill with our breathing muscles so that we can use it at a moments notice if for some reason we are put under intense physical strain. It will also make our qigong more effective as it allows us to take deeper and longer breaths and massages our internal organs more effectively due to the greater movement.

Breathing Exercise Four: Accentuated Natural Breathing

I refer to this as Accentuated Natural Breathing because while it is a natural breathing pattern and it is good for us to breathe in this way, the pattern will generally not be as obvious in our day to day activities until we begin to exert very hard, or perform qigong or other deep breathing activities. When we perform it as an exercise we emphasis each phase of the breath, or 'accentuate' it.

For this exercise, again assume a comfortable position whether sitting, kneeling, standing or lying down. Place one hand on your belly, the other on your chest so that you can more easily feel the expansion and contraction of the different parts of your body.

As you inhale through your nose, let your belly extend outwards. As you continue to inhale, draw your belly inwards as your chest expands and rises. As you exhale, let your chest fall and your belly draw back inwards.

Repeat for several inhalations and exhalations to get the feel of this type of breathing. This is an excellent type of breathing to practice for several minutes as a meditation.

__Tip:__ Getting the co-ordination right for this type of breathing can be a challenge for some people to begin with. The overall purpose of this exercise is to utilize your full breathing capacity. This means taking a full breath IN and ALSO a full breath OUT. If you do not breathe all the way out, stale air is left in the lungs; only so much additional fresh air will be able to be breathed in on top of this. Also when we breathe ALL the way out, our belly will naturally want to draw in as the diaphragm rises, then when we breathe in again the belly will naturally extend out as the diaphragm descends. This can be a great help in developing the proper co-ordination and in increasing the range of motion of the breathing muscles.

So far in these breathing exercises we have focused on placing the hands on the front of the body to feel the different parts of the body expanding and contracting. This is a good way to start as it is the front of the body that expands and contracts most, and the movement is most obvious here; ideally though, the expansion and contraction will occur on both the front and back of the body. If you lie flat on your front, ideally as you inhale, a wave of motion will move up your body, beginning as the sacrum rises followed by the lower back, mid back, upper back, neck and then ending at the head. As you breathe out this wave travels down the body in the opposite direction. This movement stimulates all of the nerves coming out from the spine. This is one of the benefits of breathing deeply and fully.

For many of us though, because of breathing and postural habits we have developed over the years, our backs have become stiff and this motion does not occur. The next exercise is a simple exercise to help stretch and loosen the muscles of the back in conjunction with the breathing.

Breathing Exercise Five: Loosening the Back

For this exercise you will need to assume a specific position. Kneel down with the tops of your feet flat on the floor. Sit your buttocks on your feet. Lean your head forward until it comes to rest on the floor. Relax your arms back by your sides. This is called the pose of the child in yoga.

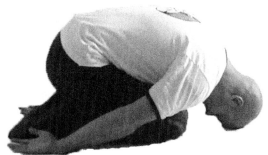

Pose of the child

Just relax and breathe deeply and fully in this position. If your back is tight, you will feel your muscles stretching as you inhale and exhale. Over time your muscles will loosen, your breathing will become easier and the movement of your spine will increase with each breath. You can stay breathing like this in this position for five minutes or more. If you want to you can also practice Breathing Exercise Three: 'Developing Skill with the Breathing Muscles' in this position.

Practicing each of these exercises will greatly increase your breathing skill, making it easier to integrate full natural relaxed breathing into your qigong practice.

There are some basic principles to follow with your breathing when doing the qigong exercises in the last section of this book. Firstly the most important thing is that your breathing needs to be deep, relaxed and slow. Breathe at a pace that is comfortable for you. Do not make your breathing too slow to begin with; it will naturally get slower and deeper with time. Also do not worry too much if you are moving your belly in and out exactly correctly, just relax and enjoy the exercises, you will improve with time. You will synchronize your movements with your breath. As a general rule you will breathe out as you make movements away from the centre of your body, and breathe in as you make movements towards the centre of your body. Specific directions for breathing are included with each exercise.

Curl your tongue up so that the tip of the tongue rests on the soft palate throughout all of the exercises. This is important for the energy circulation in your body. To find the soft palate, put the tip of your tongue behind your upper teeth. Stroke your tongue backwards, you will feel the top of your mouth is quite hard to begin with and then becomes soft. This is the soft palate where you want to leave your tongue during your exercises. This may feel awkward to begin with but will become easier with time.

As you begin to use deep, full, natural breaths in conjunction with the qigong exercises, the power of your breathing will help to subtly stretch your body throughout the movements and guide the energy through your body.

Chapter Five: Posture

In order for the energy to flow freely through our bodies, we must have good posture. Wherever there is excessive tension in our bodies or the joints are closed and not supported properly, pressure comes onto the nerves and the blood flow is restricted. As a result the energy of the body is blocked, more effort is required to maintain the position, and fatigue sets in more quickly.

Your qigong practice will help you to create good postural habits and make you very aware of the positioning of your body and when you are creating excess tension for yourself. By practicing qigong your movements will become more efficient, causing less wear and tear on your body, leaving you with more energy for the things you want to do. Finally by releasing tension from your body, your qi will be able to flow more freely, resulting in greater health and vitality.

There are a number of important principles within traditional qigong practices that will help you to achieve this. The first of these is static stance training. In this training, basic postures are held for extended periods of time. Traditionally many masters would require their students to spend months simply standing in various stances before they would begin to teach them anything else. This is because spending a long time in a position allows us to feel where we are holding tension in that posture. In order for the muscles to maintain their energy and strength, there must be a constant nervous stimulation, a flow of blood, and of qi. As the muscles begin to tire, the areas that are tight begin to become sore, the areas that do not have a good supply of nervous stimulation, blood or qi, become tired and weak and may even lose sensation. This acts as a feedback mechanism for us, we can gradually and subtly alter our posture over time so that it becomes easier and easier for us to maintain the postures. Our joints will naturally line up better to support our body and allow energy and resources to circulate. With time this will become a habit and we will begin to naturally assume mechanically sound and strong postures throughout our daily activities.

We will look at several basic postures you can practice in this way.

Horse Stance

This is a posture that you will encounter throughout the qigong exercises. It is called the horse stance because it should feel like you are sitting on the back of a horse. It may feel a little awkward and your legs – particularly your thighs will become tired to begin with, but it will become comfortable and strong with time and practice. The stance can be assumed in either a high or low position. Start with a high posture to begin with and make the posture lower as your legs become stronger and you become more comfortable in it. Either way the principles are the same.

The basic principles of this stance are:

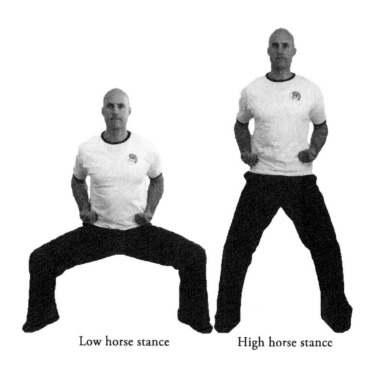

Low horse stance   High horse stance

- The feet face forward, at least hip width apart.
- The lower legs are vertical, meaning the knee is directly above the foot. The knee never extends beyond the toes.
- The pelvis is tucked under – as if you were sitting on the edge of a stool. This allows the body to move freely from the waist and takes pressure off the nerves which come out from the lower back.
- The head is held high, with the chin slightly tucked – as if suspended by a string from the center of the head.
- The shoulders are relaxed and open. One way the Chinese use to describe this is "as if you are carrying an egg under each arm." You can give this a try, it helps to have an open feeling under the shoulders

rather than being collapsed forwards or strained
backwards.

- The fists are drawn back in line with the body.

Bow Stance

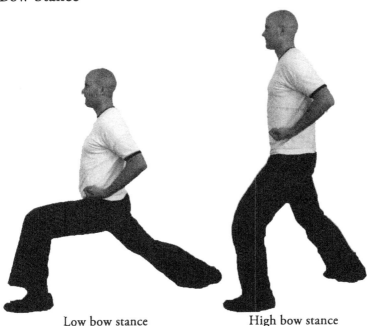

Low bow stance   High bow stance

The other basic stance you will encounter often in your
qigong practice is a Bow stance. This stance is used a lot as
we transition our weight from one leg to another and change
the direction our body is facing. Again the stance can be high
or low depending on your personal comfort levels.

The basic principles of this stance are:

- One foot is in front of the other.
- The front foot faces directly forwards.

- The knee is above the foot of the leg in front.
- The rear foot faces out to the side at around 45 degrees.
- The pelvis faces forward.
- The fists are drawn back in line with the body.

Iron Cross

Many of us have tight shoulders and a tendency to either hunch or slouch them. This posture helps to address this.

The basic principles of this posture are:

- Feet are parallel and at least shoulder width apart.
- The legs are relaxed.
- The pelvis is tucked under – as if you were sitting on a stool. This allows the body to move freely from the waist and takes pressure off the nerves emanating from the lower back.
- The head is held high with the chin slightly tucked – as if suspended by a string from the center of the head.
- The arms extend to the sides of the body at shoulder height, reaching outwards.

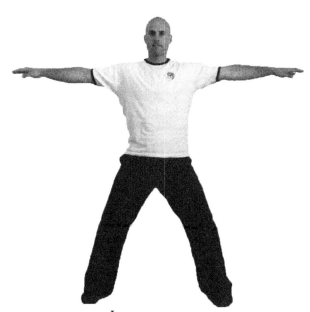

Iron cross posture

You do not need to spend months on these stances, but it pays to put some time and attention into becoming comfortable in them. Even if you only spend five minutes in each stance once a week, you will quickly become aware of the areas that become tense. With each breath in, your whole body stretches and expands subtly, relaxing as you breathe out. Over time this will cause your postures to improve, making it easier and more comfortable for you to spend longer periods of time in each of them. Your joints will open and you will begin to feel the energy circulating in your body as you relax into the stances.

Having practiced these static exercises, you will have developed good, strong, structurally sound, and balanced postures which allow your energy to flow. This is an excellent start. Achieving this will help you to achieve the same result (energy flow) as you practice the twelve moving qigong exercises at the end of this book. Eventually we want to apply these same principles to all our movements as we go about our daily activities.

Chapter Six: Awareness of Energy

The most significant benefits of the qigong exercises are the development and circulation of energy or qi in the body. The sooner you become aware of this energy and able to actually feel it, the faster you will progress.

There are many different sensations associated with qi flow. The most common are either a magnetic feeling as if either two opposite poles of a magnet are pulling together or two same poles are pushing apart, or a feeling of warmth, or both. Sometimes people also describe sensations of tingling or a breeze on the skin. As you progress with your practice of qigong you will feel all of these sensations and probably others too. You may start to feel these sensations straight away, or it may take you awhile. Whatever the case, just accept what you feel, there is no use trying to convince yourself you are feeling something you aren't. Keep practicing and it will come in time. Once you feel something, even just a tiny sensation, you can begin to grow it. You can direct your mind to send more energy into an area and increase the sensation and your awareness.

Initially you will probably be most aware of the energy in your hands. This is because we are used to being quite aware of our hands, using them to feel things, using them for activities that require fine motor control and awareness. Our hands are rich with nerve endings and the blood flows to them easily. Over time as you continue to practice, the flow of energy will increase and you will begin to feel these sensations up your arms and eventually over the rest of your body and legs.

The following exercises will help you to develop your initial qi awareness.

Simple exercise to become aware of Qi

Clap you hands together vigorously in a random intermittent pattern for at least one minute. At the end of this your hands will feel warm and maybe a little tingly. This is good. The clapping stimulates the nerve endings in the hands and brings a rush of blood into the area. The flow of qi is closely related to the functioning of our nervous system and the flow of blood in our bodies.

Bring your hands close together in front of you, but not touching. You should be able to feel the warmth between your hands from the clapping.

Now begin to move your hands in and out, just slightly, bringing your hands closer together and further apart. Only move them as far as you can while still feeling the warm sensation between your hands.

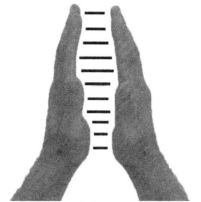

Feel the warmth between your hands

As you practice this keep moving your hands further apart.
In time you will also feel the beginnings of a magnetic pull or
push between your hands as you move them. As you move
your hands further apart, imagine you are squeezing a warm
ball of magnetic energy as you move your hands together, and
it pushes back against your hands as you move your hands
apart.

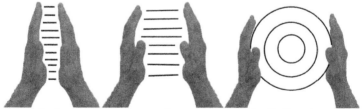

Move the hands further apart then together again feeling the energy

Remember to breathe!

In my experience about 75% of people begin to feel qi in
their first attempt at this exercise. Those who do not should
persist and they will feel it in time.

This exercise is a good one to do on a regular basis along with the health exercises, to increase your awareness and control of qi.

Pulling a string

Standing in a relaxed position.

Imagine there is a ring on the floor in front of you between your feet.

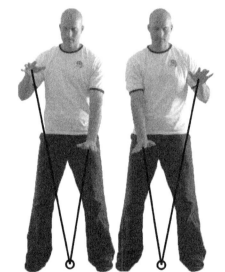

Imagine a piece of string or column of energy

There is a string that passes through the ring and is tied to the middle finger of each of your hands.

As you lift your right hand, the left is pulled down towards the ring. As you raise the left hand, the right hand is pulled down towards the ring.

42

Move your hands up and down feeling the pull on your other hand.

This exercise can also be done, imagining that instead of a string, there is a column of energy extending from one hand down to a point on the floor and back up to your other hand. As you push down on the column of energy with one hand, the other hand is pushed up.

Pushing against a wall

Standing fairly close to a wall, raise both hands in front of you.

Start to move your hands closer and further away from the wall.

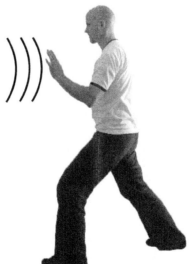

Feel the energy in your push

As you do this, feel the magnetic energy compressing and pushing back against your hands.

Rolling around a ball of energy

Bring your hands together until you begin to feel a ball of energy between them.

Begin to move the hands in a circular motion as if rubbing around the edges of a ball.
Allow the hands to move further apart as you maintain your awareness of this sensation of rubbing your hands across the surface of a ball.

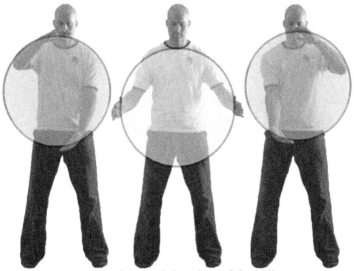

Feel around the edges of the ball

Once the ball has expanded as far as you wish it to, begin to squeeze it back together as you continue to move your hands in a circular motion. As you do this you may feel the heat intensify between your hands, the magnetic feeling may increase, the ball may begin to feel quite heavy.

Chapter Seven: Chinese Medicine Concepts

Chinese medicine has a long and rich history dating back thousands of years; for millennia it has proven to be effective in treating a wide range of different ailments. Today many people still use it as their primary form of healthcare for all but the most acute and severe ailments - when western medical options such as refined pharmaceuticals and surgical procedures are sought. Often Chinese medicine will yield results when western medicine has no answers, particularly in chronic conditions, or difficult to diagnose cases.

Part of the reason for Chinese and Western medicine's differing capacities to deal with particular types of health problems is that Chinese medicine and Western medicine developed along quite different lines with quite different underlying philosophies. Early on Western medical practitioners and researchers started to use dissection as a primary tool for understanding the body and its functions. Consequently Western medicine has placed strong emphasis on the physical structures of the body, and treatment often focuses on individual structures. This approach has many advantages and led to the development of sophisticated surgical procedures and extremely potent pharmaceutical products with very specific focused actions.

The Chinese on the other hand did not place nearly as much emphasis on dissection, focusing instead on observation of the living organism from the outside. This led to a sophisticated understanding of the interactive nature of the systems in the human body, and an understanding of how the mind influences the functioning of the body. As such, Chinese medical philosophy focuses not so much on the physical structures of the body as on functional groupings within the body and how they influence each other.

Early on they came up with the concept of 'qi' or 'energy' as a way to understand and explain these groupings and interactions. This 'qi' or energy circulates throughout the body, regulating the function of every organ and every cell. Understanding the flow of qi leads to a subtle understanding of the functioning of the body, giving rise to different options for treatment and health maintenance.

Qi has not yet been well defined in western scientific terms, but it has been measured by scientists in terms of differences in electrical resistance, thermal radiation of specific wavelengths and even as sound energy at certain frequencies. Research in this area is ongoing and we can look forward to exciting developments in the future as Western and Chinese medical thought begins to converge.

The main pathways the qi flows along are referred to as meridians. There are twelve major meridians in the body, each associated with an internal organ and group of functions in the body. In addition to this there are what are referred to as 'Dantien' or 'fields of elixir', where the body stores qi for use in the future.

The Dantien

There are several dantien or elixir fields throughout the body. They act as storage areas for the body's qi. One of these dantien is of such importance that often people will refer to it simply as 'The Dantien'. We will restrict our discussion to this dantien at this stage.

The dantien is located a few inches below the navel and deep in the centre of the body. As you progress with the exercises in this book you will want to become more and more aware of this area and the energy stored there. It is very important to correctly locate your dantien with your mind. A common mistake is to mentally place it on the surface of your body. Thinking about it as just in front of your spine will help you to correctly locate the right area.

From a western perspective we know several things about this area that help us to understand why the dantien is so important.

1. It is the natural centre of gravity of our physical bodies. One of the energies we work with throughout our life is that of weight and gravity, or kinetic energy. When our bodies are well aligned, all the kinetic energy we are subjected to will transmit through our dantien. Our whole body will function as one unit, sharing the load and strains evenly. When we are not well aligned, our dantien will not be in the centre of our body and some parts of our body will have to compensate for others, putting excessive strain on joints, muscles and connective tissue. We will also feel off-balance. You may have heard people say, if when you are trying to stand on one

leg and having a hard time maintaining your balance, you put the finger of one hand on your belly button, this will help you. This works, and it is because the belly button is close to our centre of gravity. By putting your finger there, you are also putting part of your awareness there and helping to organize your body around your centre of gravity. When we put our awareness at our dantien we are doing something similar, helping to balance and distribute all the physical forces we are subject to throughout our bodies.

2. This area is in the midst of our digestive tract surrounded by our intestines which are responsible for absorbing nutrients from the food we eat and for producing things like vitamin B-12 which has a large role in how energetic we feel. Putting our awareness in this area helps to stimulate our digestion. You may notice your tummy gurgling as you practice qigong, or with practice you may notice a warm sensation building up in this area.

3. When we breathe, if our primary breathing muscle—our diaphragm, is working properly, this area will expand as we inhale and the diaphragm descends, and then contract as we continue to inhale and the ribcage expands. It will then expand as the ribcage relaxes again and contract again as the diaphragm raises back up. This is a lot of movement, and tension in the area of our dantien can stop this from occurring properly. By putting our awareness there we help to relax the area and regulate this movement, allowing our breath to function more efficiently.

4. The dantien is also located in the midst of the enteric nervous system. This is an interesting branch of the human nervous system comprising 200-600 million neurons. This is

about the same number as is contained in the entire spinal cord. The enteric nervous system is also unique in that is has complete circuits within it. In a very real way it can 'think' autonomously from the central nervous system and brain. Has anyone ever told you to listen to a gut feeling? Sometimes your gut can actually figure things out before your brain does! It also contains many two-way connections with the central nervous system, so passes information and signals on to the rest of the body. This area is a hive of electrical activity and so is an important centre of electrical energy in the body.

The dantien will be one of your first points of mental focus as you carry out the exercises in this book. It is also helpful to bring your awareness back to your dantien at the end of each qigong session to help you move into the rest of your day with your energy centered and balanced.

The Major Meridians

As mentioned earlier, each of these meridians is associated with an internal organ in the body. It is important to remember though, that the meridians do not deal solely with the physical structure of that organ but with a whole set of functions throughout the body. As such the meridians extend from the tips of the fingers right down to the soles of the feet. Also two of the meridians associate with structures we do not typically think of as organs. These are the Circulation Sex or Pericardium and Triple Warmer meridians.

The twelve exercises contained in this book are designed to stimulate the flow of qi in each of the major meridians through gentle stretching and compression, or in other words massage. You will notice this as you perform the exercises with an awareness of the related organ and its meridian.

Each meridian is more active at a certain time of day than at others. During this time, the related organ and functions are being repaired and maintained by the body. Because of this, different meridians and organs are more susceptible to influence at different times. For this reason the exercises are performed in a specific order in harmony with the sequence the energy naturally flows through the body. The exercise you begin the sequence with is the exercise that relates to the meridian that is currently at its peak level of activity, as this is where the energy is (or should) already be flowing strongly. So the exercise you begin the series with will vary depending on what time of day you are practicing. You then continue with the rest of the exercises in sequential order of peak activity. By performing the exercises in this way we help to keep our bodies in harmony with the natural cycles of the world around us.

Charts which show the twelve internal organs and their meridians follow. Each meridian pathway is quite complex, each has many internal connections and sections which branch off the main pathways. They also travel a three dimensional path, coming closer to the surface at some points and descending deeper at others. This is difficult to represent in a two dimensional images. It is also very difficult for a beginning qigong practitioner to conceptualize and follow with their mind.

What is shown in the charts are simplified pathways. These show only the main branches of each meridian. While there is actually more to the meridians, following the pathways represented in the charts with your mind will be sufficient to stimulate the flow of energy through the entire meridian and its branches.

Gallbladder
Peak activity: 11pm – 1am

This meridian begins near the corner of the eye and finishes on the outside edge of the fourth toe. The organ sits under the liver on the right hand side of the body

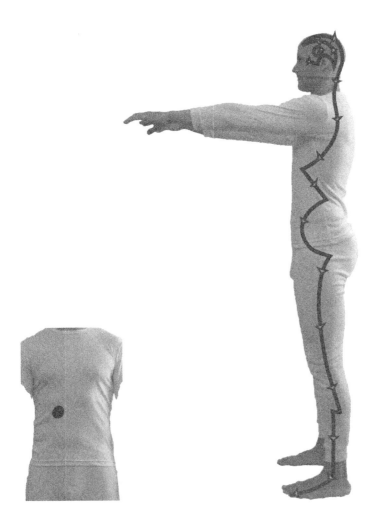

Liver
Peak activity: 1am – 3am

This meridian begins on the top of the big toe and ends below the sixth rib. The organ sits under the ribs, mainly on the right side.

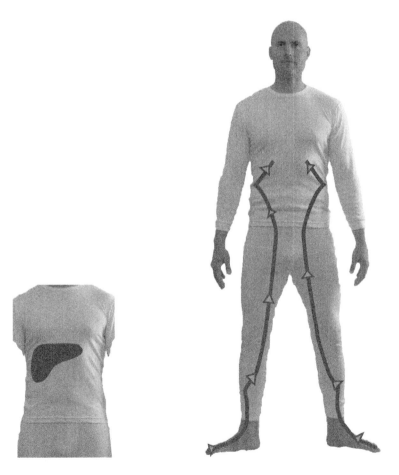

Lungs
Peak activity: 3am – 5am

This meridian begins in the joint of the shoulder and ends on the tip of the thumb. The organ sits behind the ribs on either side of the sternum.

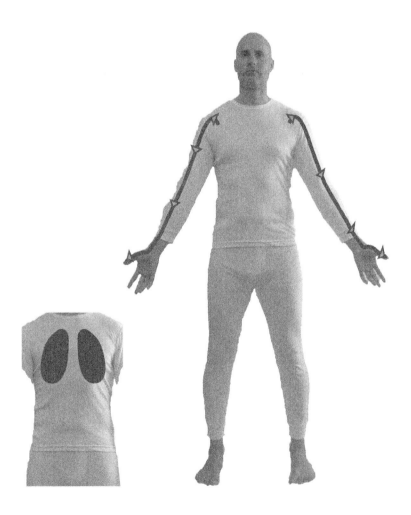

Large Intestine
Peak activity: 5am – 7am

This meridian begins on the tip of the index finger and ends just below the nose on the face. The organ makes a circuit around the lower portion of the torso in a clockwise direction.

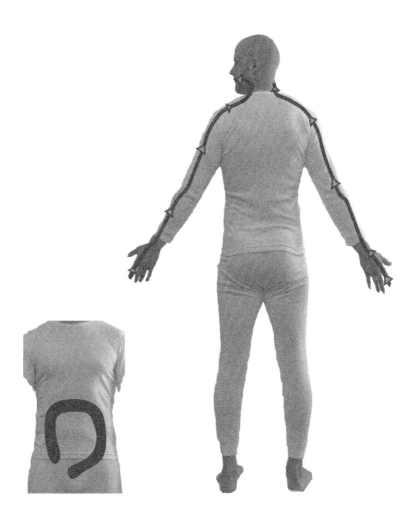

Stomach

Peak activity: 7am – 9am

This meridian begins just below the eye and ends on the second toe. The organ is in the centre of the body and slightly to the left.

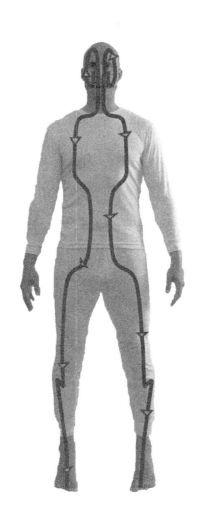

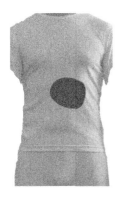

Spleen

Peak activity: 9am – 11am

This meridian begins on the inside of the big toe and ends alongside the 6th rib. The organ is in the midline of the body to the left of the stomach, under the ribs.

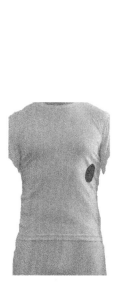

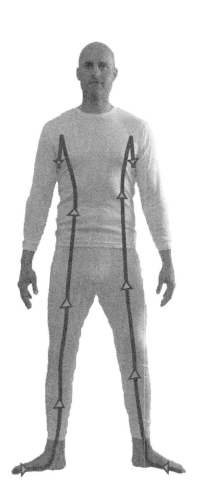

Heart

Peak activity: 11am – 1pm

This meridian begins deep in the armpit and ends on the inside of the little finger. The organ is in the centre of the chest, behind the sternum and slightly to the left.

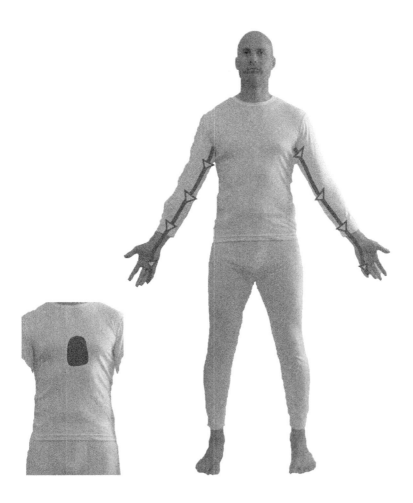

Small Intestine

Peak activity: 1pm – 3pm

This meridian begins on the outside of the little finger and
ends just in front of the ear. The organ is located in the
centre of the lower portion of the abdomen.

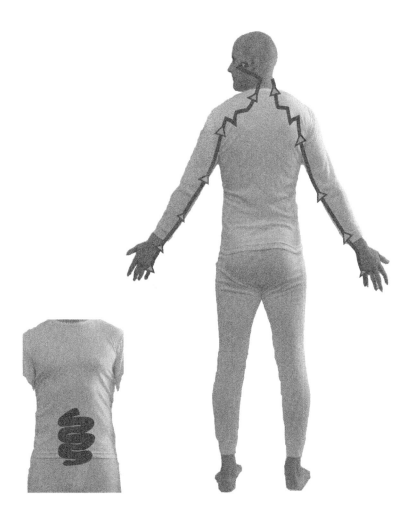

Bladder

Peak activity: 3pm – 5pm

This meridian begins above the eye and ends on the outside of the little toe. The organ is located at the centre of the bottom of the abdomen.

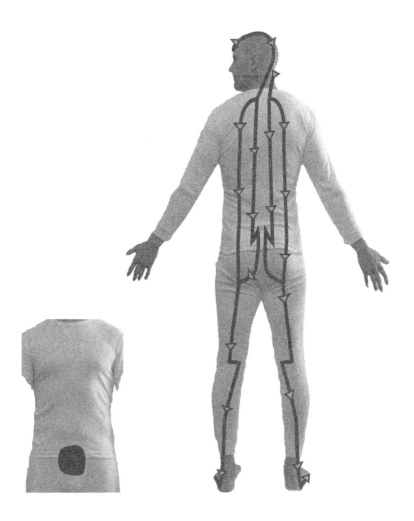

Kidneys
Peak activity: 5pm – 7pm

This meridian begins on the sole of the foot, just behind the ball of the foot. It ends just below the collar bone. The organs are located at the rear of the torso in the lower back.

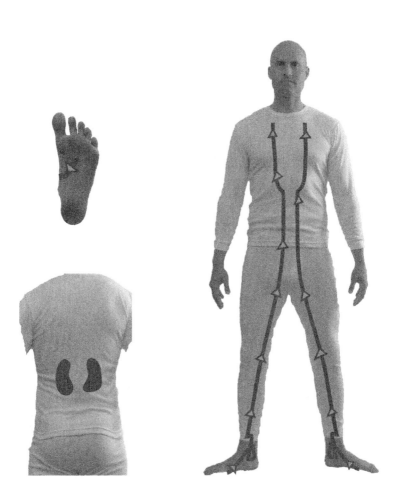

Circulation Sex or Pericardium

Peak activity: 7pm – 9pm

This meridian begins beside the nipple and ends on the side of the middle finger. The organ consists of the lining of each of the other organs, so is spread through the entire torso.

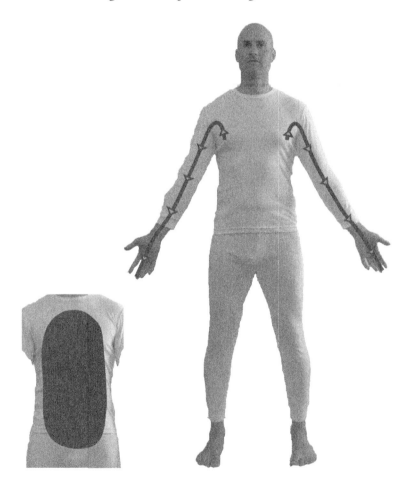

Triple Warmer

Peak activity: 9pm – 11pm

This meridian begins on the outside of the fourth finger and ends on the temple. The organ is the space that each of the other organs sits within, so surrounds the entire torso.

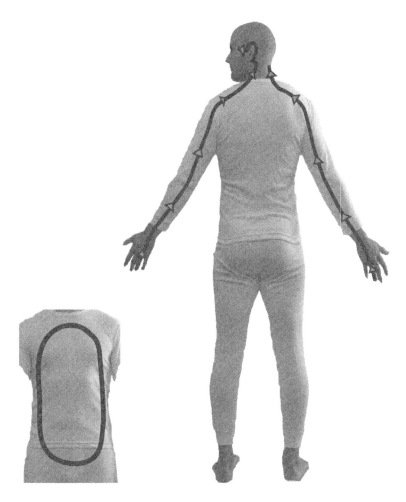

Chapter Eight: Practicing the exercises

As has been mentioned in earlier chapters, qigong is as much about the mind as it is the body. Whenever we begin a qigong session we will go through a checklist of:

1. Quieting the mind and directing the intention.
2. Correct posture to allow free movement of energy.
3. Regulating the breath to stimulate the energy and influence the body.
4. Awareness of energy

Levels of Awareness

The exercises have benefits on numerous levels. Each exercise works, stretches and loosens muscles and joints throughout the body, helps to integrate our breath with our movements, develops and stores energy in the dantien – balancing the body in relation to gravity and the kinetic forces of the movement, internally massages an organ and the nerves leading to that organ, and finally - stimulates the flow of energy through the meridian related to that organ. For this reason there are different levels of awareness of energy as you practice these exercises. These are:

- Awareness of the sensation of the muscles, joints and spine as the movements are performed
- Awareness of the stretching and releasing effect the breath has on the movement
- Awareness of the dantien

- Awareness of the organ being internally massaged
- Awareness of energy flow in the related meridian

It is best if you begin by learning just a couple of exercises at a time. Practice these until you a very comfortable with them and how the movements feel to you. Continue to add one or two of the exercises to your practice sessions until you know all twelve and are comfortable with the sensations in your muscles, joints and spine as your perform them.

Now begin to put greater awareness on your breath and the stretching and releasing effect each has throughout the movements. Synchronize the breath with the movement. Exhaling as the limbs move away from the center of the body and inhaling as they move towards the center.
Next add to this awareness of the dantien and how the body expands and contracts around this point.

When you begin to work on awareness of the organ being internally massaged it becomes important to perform the exercises in the correct sequence according to the time of day. These times are included on both the meridian charts and the instructions for each exercise.

Finally, add to this awareness of the energy moving along the related meridian. This will probably be quite subtle at first, but will grow stronger with practice. You will want to refer back to the charts of the meridians in the previous chapter for this.

Remember: it is not a race. Take your time with each of these steps, making sure you master each one in turn. You will gain more benefit in this way than by jumping ahead and trying to have all the focuses straight away. This will probably take you several months.

The exercises are designed to be performed slowly with the absolute minimum tension in all of the movements and positions. The more slowly you perform the exercises, the more benefit you will get. Do not force yourself to go slower than you are comfortable with though. Allow yourself to slow down gradually as you progress. Performing the exercises slowly will allow you time to develop the energy awareness which is so important to qigong practice.

Remember this point when you are conducting your qigong practice sessions. Do not try to rush through a particular number of repetitions of the exercises. See how much time you have available for your session and judge how many times you will be able to comfortably repeat each exercise at a leisurely pace. Even doing each exercise just once will stimulate the energy throughout your whole system and provide you with great benefit.

Seated Position

If you have difficulty performing the exercises standing, with minor modifications you can perform them sitting down instead. Ideally you will do this sitting on the edge of a stool at a height that puts your thighs roughly parallel with the ground, as this helps to maintain the optimum posture through the spine for these exercises.

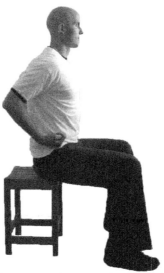

Performing qigong exercises seated on the edge of a stool.

This is also an excellent way to improve your posture in the horse stance. Performing the exercises in this way intensifies the stretching effect they have on the spine; this will help to release your lower back muscles, making it easier to stand in a horse stance with your pelvis tucked under.

If a stool such as this is not available, or you find this uncomfortable, you can try the exercises seated in another type of chair.

Qi Locks

In some of the exercises the hands assume specific shapes known at 'qi locks'. These hand shapes are designed to help keep the energy circulating within the body rather than being sent out from the body. Whenever we form a fist in the qigong exercises, we put our thumb inside the fingers like so:

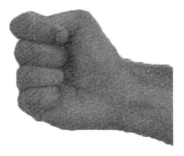

Qi lock with thumb inside fist.

Never punch someone like this – you will break your thumb; it is a useful fist for energy development though, as many meridians end in the tips of the fingers. By turning each of them, including the thumb, into the centre of the palm we help to re-circulate and build up the supply of energy in our bodies.

The other qi lock you will encounter in these exercises looks like this:

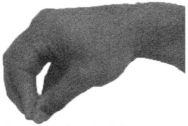

Crane's head qi lock with all fingertips touching.

This qi lock is called the crane's head. All five fingertips are brought together so they touch each other facilitating the free circulation of qi.

Your Qigong Session

It is recommended that you conduct your qigong session in the following order:

1. Warm up
2. The twelve exercises
3. Cool down

1. The warm up involves gently rotating each of the major joints in the body. This provides an opportunity for you to quiet your mind and bring your attention away from whatever you have been thinking about or working on and focus on your body. These movements will help to lubricate the joints and make sure everything is moving freely before you begin the twelve exercises. Be aware of any areas that are stiff or sore and gently relax these areas and send energy to them in preparation for the exercises.

2. The exercises should be performed in order according to the time of day you are practicing. Start with the exercise that correlates with the organ that is at peak activity levels at the time you are practicing. Continue with the rest of the exercises in the order of peak activity time, finishing again with the organ which is currently at peak activity levels.

If at any time during the exercises you become breathless, dizzy, or otherwise feel out of sorts, simply take a rest for a minute or two to let your breathing and energy normalize before returning to the exercises.

The related organ, time of day of peak activity and other general benefits of each exercise are noted with the description of the exercise.

3. Begin the cool down by placing your hands on your lower abdomen in front of the dantien. Become aware of the energy in the dantien and focus on your slow steady breathing. The cool down continues with a simple self massage routine correlating with the direction of energy flow in the meridians. You can do this by either rubbing patting, or running your hands over your body with the hands not quite touching the body in the directions indicated. This will help to distribute the energy through your entire body and leave you feeling stimulated and refreshed.

Finish the cool down by returning your hands to the lower abdomen, bringing your awareness back to your dantien and your breath for a few moments.

The Warm Up

Wrist rotation

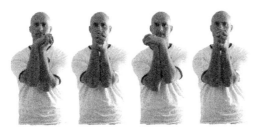

Clasp both of your hands together and rotate them several times, clockwise then anti-clockwise.

Elbow rotation

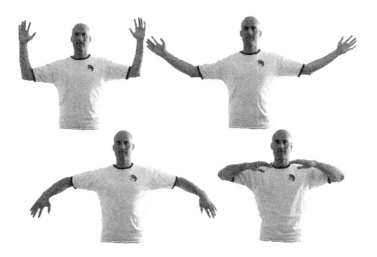

Raise your arms to your sides. Keeping your upper arms relatively still, rotate your lower arms in a circular motion several times, first one way, then the other.

Shoulder rotation

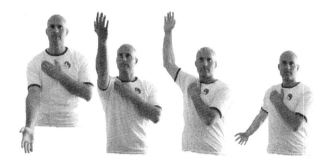

Rotate each of your arms at the shoulder several times, first backward then forward. Place your other hand so that the fingertips press into the joint of your shoulder to support this movement.

Waist rotation

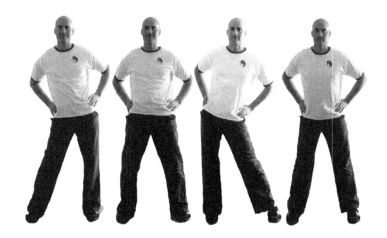

Keeping your head upright, move your hips to the side, front, other side and back in a smooth circular motion. Repeat several times in each direction.

Knee rotation

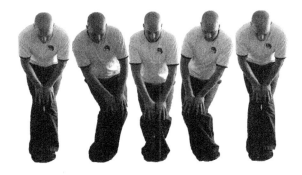

With your feet close together bend forward and rest your hands on top of your knees. Move your knees to the side, forwards, to the other side and back in a smooth circular motion several times in each direction.

Ankle rotation

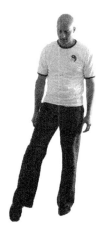

Place the toes of one of your feet on the ground. Rotate your ankle several times in each direction. Repeat with your other ankle.

Spine rotation

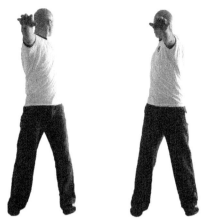

With your feet shoulder width apart, raise one arm forwardsand one arm back. Turn your head to look at your back hand. Swing your arms down by your sides then up again, switching the position of each hand. Turn your head to look at the hand that is now at the back. This gives your spine a gentle twist. Repeat in a rhythmic smooth motion several times.

The Twelve Exercises

1. Tiger Stretches it's Back

Organ: Gallbladder
Peak Activity: 11pm – 1 am

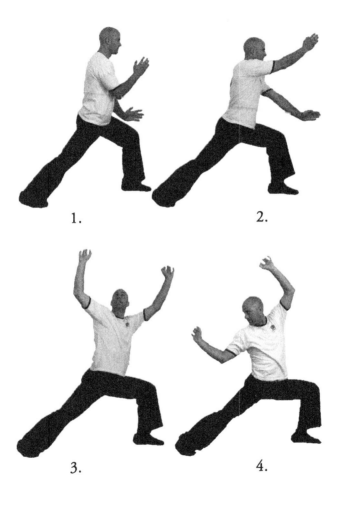

1.   2.

3.   4.

1. Inhale as you turn to your left in a bow stance with your hands in front of you, right hand high, left hand low.
2. Exhale as you sink lower into your stance and extend your arms forward.
3. Continue to exhale as you reach your hands up over your head, following them with your gaze.
4. Finish looking towards the rear.

Inhale as you turn to your right and repeat the sequence of movements in this direction.

2. Four Body Movements

Organ: Liver
Peak Activity: 1am – 3am

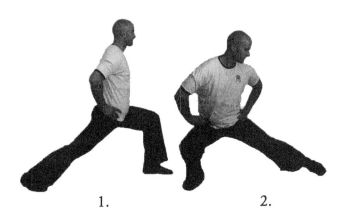

1.   2.

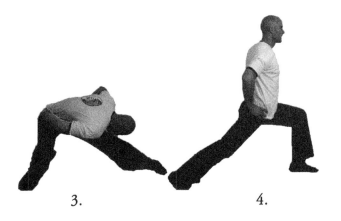

3.   4.

1. Exhale as you turn and lunge out to your left side in a bow stance.
2. Inhale as you sit your weight back onto your right leg.
3. Exhale as you lean your body down towards your left leg, keeping your pelvis above your right leg.
4. Continue to exhale as you lunge forwards again with your weight over your left leg.

Continue to exhale as you turn and assume a bow stance facing to your right. Repeat the sequence of movements in this direction.

3. Dragon Clears a Path

Organ: Lungs
Peak Activity: 3am – 5am

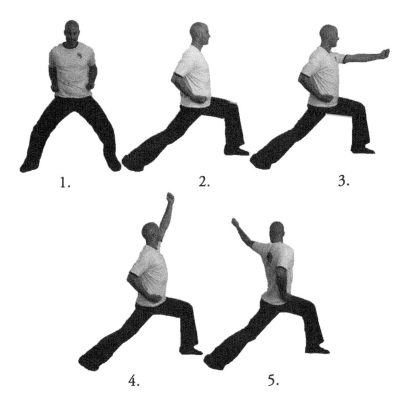

1. Standing in a horse stance, inhale as you draw your fists back in line with your waist.
2. Turn to your left - assuming a bow stance.
3. Exhale as you extend your left fist out from your centre.
4. Inhale as you begin to raise your extended left arm.

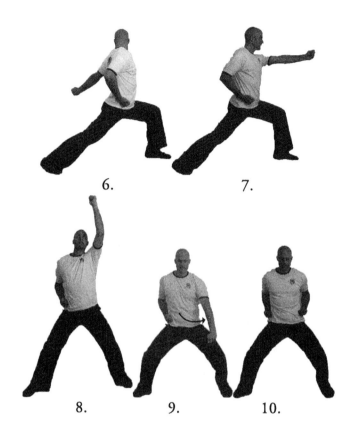

6.   7.

8.   9.   10.

5-7. Continue to inhale as you follow your fist with your gaze, making a complete circle behind your body.

8. Continue to inhale as you raise your fist directly above your head as you turn you body forwards.

9. Exhale as you bring your arm down in front of your body in a semi – circle.

10. Inhale as you bring your fists back in line with your body. Repeat with your right arm, facing the other direction.

4. Bending the Body and Swinging the Head

Organ: Large Intestine
Peak Activity: 5am – 7am

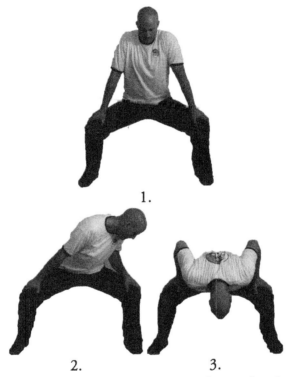

1.

2.   3.

1. Sink down into a low horse stance with your hands resting on your knees.
2-5. Inhale as you bring your body down towards the left, centre, and then upwards on the right - returning to the starting position. Make as large a circle a can with your head. Support the weight of your body on your arms which are resting on your knees.
6-8. Repeat in the other direction as you exhale.

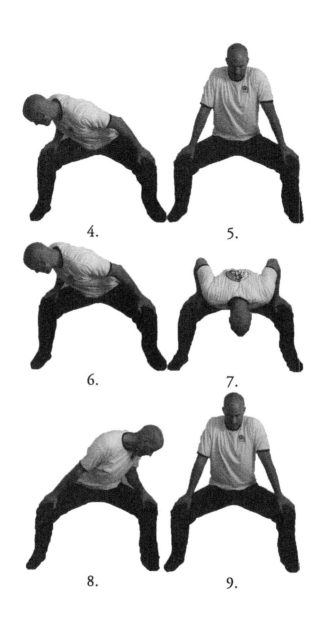

4.   5.

6.   7.

8.   9.

After completing this, repeat the entire sequence inhaling to the right and exhaling to the left.

5. One Arm Raising

Organ: Stomach
Peak Activity: 7am – 9am

1.   2.   3.   4.

5.   6.

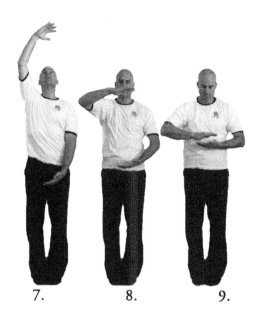

7.   8.   9.

1. Begin with your feet close together.
2. Inhale as you bring your palms together, left hand on top of right.
3. Exhale as you extend your left hand up and right hand down. Raise up on your toes at the same time.
4–7. Inhale as you circle your hands in a large circle, ending with your right hand high and left hand low.
8–9. Continue to inhale as you bring your palms close together, right hand above left. Lower down of your toes back onto flat feet.

Repeat in the other direction by exhaling as you extend your right hand high and left hand low. Circle your hands in the opposite direction as you inhale.

6. Crane Looks Behind

Organ: Spleen
Peak activity: 9am – 11am

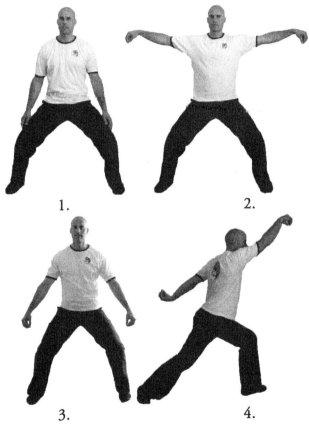

1.   2.

3.   4.

1-4. Inhale as you raise your arms to shoulder level, lower
   your arms to your sides and turn out to the left raising
   your right arm forwards and left arm backwards. Turn
   your feet so that each faces outwards at a 45 degree angle
   (left foot 45 degrees to the left, right foot 45 degrees to the
   right).

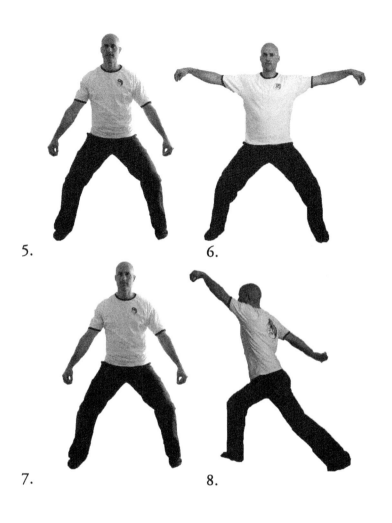

5.

6.

7.

8.

5-8. Exhale as you perform the same movements turning out
   to your right.

Repeat the entire sequence, inhaling as you turn to the right
and exhaling as you turn to the left.

7. Wild Goose Beats it's Wings

Organ: Heart
Peak activity: 11am – 1pm

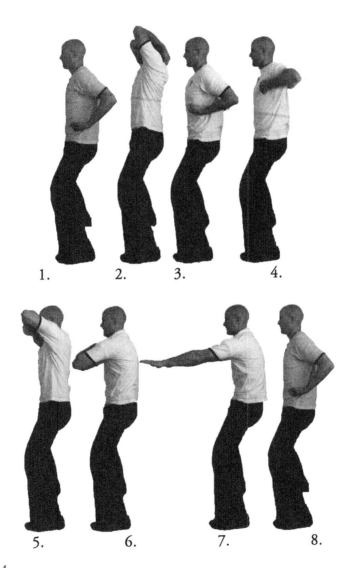

1. 2. 3. 4.

5. 6. 7. 8.

1. Inhale as you draw your fists back in line with your body.
2. Exhale as you raise your elbows up.
3. Continue to exhale as you draw your elbows backwards again.
4-5. Continue to exhale as you roll your elbows up and forwards in a circular motion.
6. End this circular motion with your elbows pointing directly to the front.
7. Continue to exhale as you extend your arms forwards, fingers extended.
8. Inhale as you draw your fists back in line with your waist.

8. *Punching Wind.*

Organ: Small Intestine
Peak activity: 1pm – 3pm

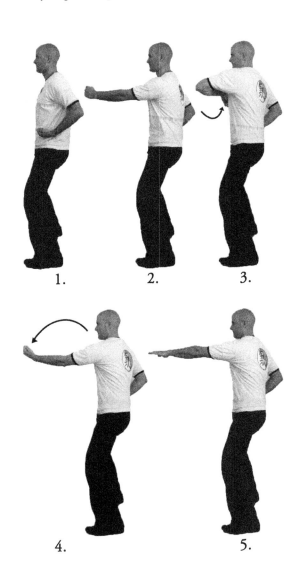

1.   2.   3.

4.   5.

1. Inhale as you draw your fists back in line with your waist.
2. Exhale, extending your left fist forward from your centre.
3. Continue to exhale as you lower the fist, drawing it back towards you in a circular motion, keeping your elbow pointing forward.
4. Continue to exhale as you extend the back of your fist forward in a circular motion.
5. Continue to exhale as you turn your hand over and extend your fingers.

Finish the movement by inhaling as you draw your fist back in line with your waist. Repeat with your other arm.

9. Black Tiger Straightens it's Waist

Organ: Bladder
Peak activity: 3pm – 5pm

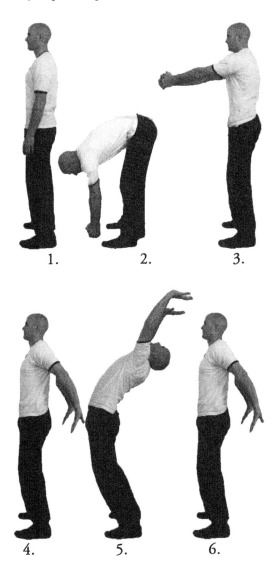

1.   2.   3.

4.   5.   6.

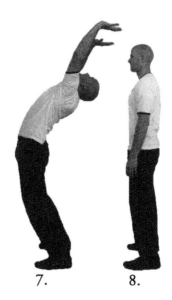

7.   8.

1. Begin with your arms at your sides.
2. Inhale bending forwards interlocking your fingers.
3. Exhale as you stand up, raising your arms till they are about level with your shoulders.
4. Inhale lowering your arms and extend them backwards.
5. Exhale as you reach your hands up and backwards over your head.
6. Continue to exhale as you lower your arms again.
7. Continue to exhale as you stretch your hands up and backwards over your head again.
8. Inhale as you lower your arms forwards and down to rest at your sides.

10. Man Riding a Horse, Drawing a Bow and Arrow

Organ: Kidneys
Peak activity: 5pm – 7pm

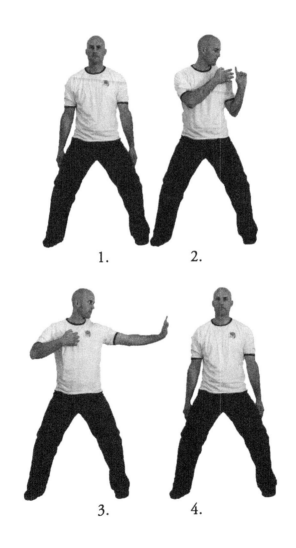

1.   2.

3.   4.

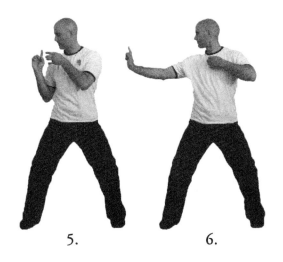

5.   6.

1. Begin with your arms by your sides.
2. Inhale as you draw your arms up so that your left hand is in front of your left shoulder, index finger extended. Your right hand is just behind the left with the fingers extended.
3. Exhale as you extend your left arm, focusing on the index finger of your left hand as if it were a bow. The right hand draws back to the centre of the chest as if it were drawing the string of the bow back.
4. Inhale as you lower your arms.
5. Continue to inhale as you raise your hands to your right side.
6. Exhale as you extend your right hand and draw the fingers of your left hand back to the centre of your chest.

11. Turning and Gazing

Organ: Circulation Sex or Pericardium
Peak activity: 7pm – 9pm

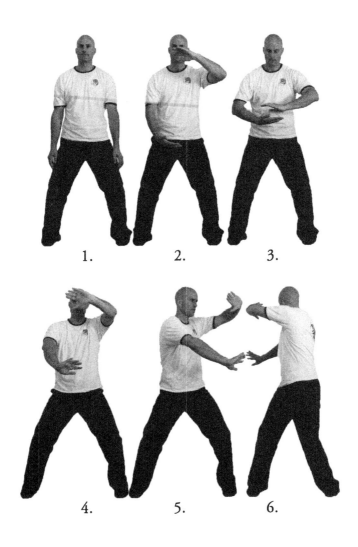

1.   2.   3.

4.   5.   6.

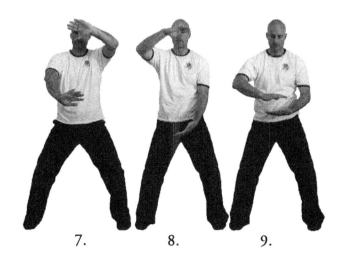

7.   8.   9.

1. Begin with your arms at your sides.
2. Inhale as you circle your hands so that your left hand is above your right.
3. Continue to inhale as you bring your hands close together.
4. Exhale, pressing your hands forwards, left hand high, right hand low.
5. Exhale as you twist left with your gaze on your left hand.
6. Continue to exhale as you twist toward the right with your gaze on the left hand.
7. Inhale as you turn back to face forwards.
8. Continue to inhale as you circle your hands around so that your right hand is now high.
9. Continue to inhale as you bring your palms close together in front of your body.

Repeat by exhaling as you press your hands forward, right hand high and left hand low, then continue to exhale as you twist to the right and then the left.

12. Two Hands Push the Sky

Organ: Triple Warmer
Peak activity: 9pm – 11pm

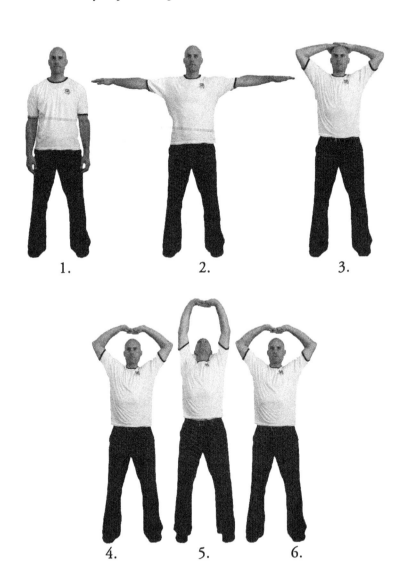

1.   2.   3.

4.   5.   6.

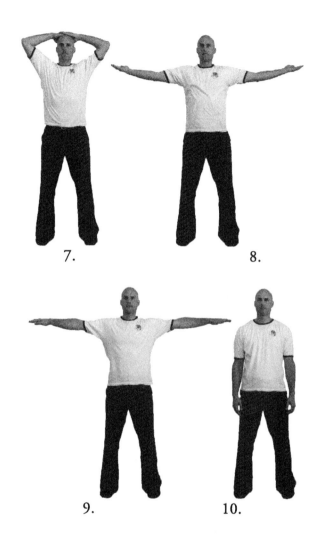

7.

8.

9.

10.

1. Begin with your hands by your sides.
2. Inhale raising your arms up by your sides.
3. Continue to inhale as you bring your hands above your head and interlock your fingers.

4. Turn your hands over so that your palms face upwards.
5. Exhale extending your hands towards the sky, looking upwards and raising up on your toes.
6. Continue to exhale as you lower your hands back towards your head.
7. Turn your hands over so the palms now face back towards your head.
8. Inhale as you lower your arms back to shoulder height.
9. Turn your palms over so they now face the ground.
10. Exhale as you lower your arms back to your sides.

The Cool Down

Energy Massage

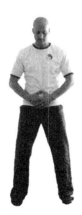

Begin with your hands resting on your lower abdomen. Take a few moments to be aware of your dantien and your breath.

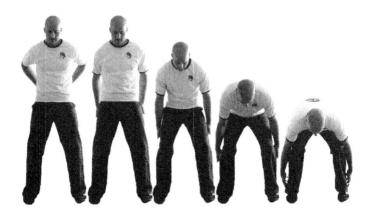

Separate your hands and bring them behind your back. Run your hands down the back outside of your legs to your feet.

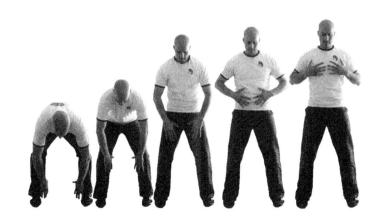

Run your hands up the inside front of your legs and body to your chest level.

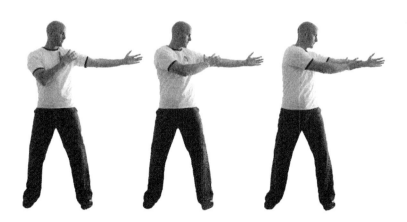

Run your right hand out the inside of your left arm, from shoulder to hand.

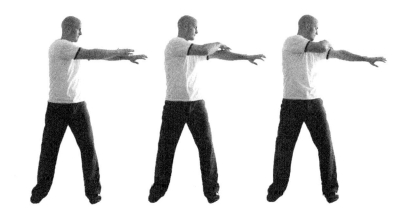

Turn your arm over and run your right hand back up the
outside of your left arm.

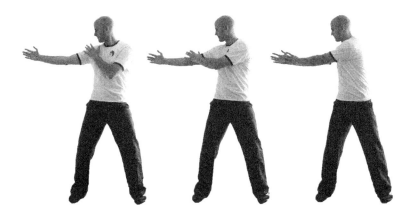

Run your left hand out the inside of your right arm from
shoulder to hand.

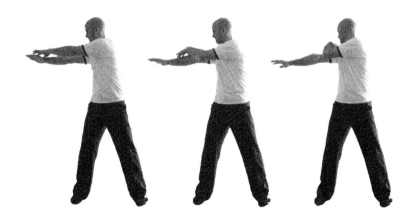

Turn your arm over and run your left hand from hand to shoulder down the back of your right arm.

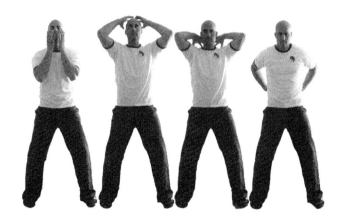

Run both hands up over your face and head, down over your shoulders and back to the back of your waist. Repeat this sequence as many times as you wish.

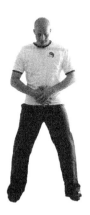

Finish by returning your hands back to your lower abdomen. Return your awareness to your dantien and your breathing.

Chapter Nine: The Path Ahead

This introductory book on qigong provides basic knowledge of qigong practices and a simple set of exercises for you to begin your practice with. For most people it will take several months to master the contents of this book. Even after years of practice, as you continue to perform these exercises you will find that you continue to learn - as you become more and more aware of your body and the subtle flow of energy within it.

Sometimes we tend to forget that the 'gong' in qigong means work. Do not expect to understand everything all at once, or to reap all the benefits after just one short burst of practice. Progress is much more likely to be slow and steady. Practice regularly and enjoy the process.

This may be as far as you wish to go in your qigong journey. If so, regular practice or what you have learnt in this book will be rewarding. The exercises in this book provide a firm base for ongoing health and wellbeing.

On the other hand it is possible you may want to delve more deeply into the world of qigong. This book has focused on a few simple introductory practices; but there is much more in terms of theory and also more complex and sophisticated practices and applications of qigong that you can explore.

If you do want to learn more, make sure that you have mastered the practices in this book first before moving on to further practice and study. Qigong is primarily about doing;

further theoretical knowledge or advanced exercises will be of little use to you without enough physical experience to support you in your learning. It may even slow down your progress as you become distracted by different ideas when you have not yet mastered the skills which are precursors to using this knowledge.

If you do wish to pursue your study of qigong further, this book is the first in a planned series of books and DVDs on the subject. Future books will examine in more depth, and provide practices related to topics such as:

- Advanced Moving Qigong Forms
- Self Healing through Qigong
- Hard Qigong
- Interacting with the energies around us – the magnetic energy of the earth, the energy of the sun and heavenly bodies and other environmental influences
- Application of Qigong to different tasks – martial arts, sports and healing

Check regularly at www.developyourqi.com for new titles. You can also sign up to an e-mail newsletter there which will keep you informed with articles about qigong and related subjects, and news about events and seminars.

Wherever your journey takes you, I hope that you have enjoyed this book and that you will use the exercises contained within it for years to come, to develop your qi, and improve and maintain your health and wellbeing throughout your life.

About the Author

John Munro has studied traditional Chinese medicine and qigong under the tutelage of Alastair Laubach-Bourne, the grandmaster of the Wah family, southern tiger style, since the year 2000. His passion is the application of qigong principles to all aspects of day to day life.

At the time of publication he serves as the secretary of the New Zealand Chi Kung and Traditional Chinese Medicine Association, and on the executive board of the New Zealand Charter of Health Practitioners.

His qualifications include:

Diploma Traditional Chinese Medicine
Diploma Chi Kung
Certified Neuro Linguistic Programmer
Certificate Remedial Massage
Certificate Personal Training

He can be contacted through his website at:

www.developyourqi.com

Printed in Great Britain
by Amazon

38291387R00076